52 Tips
for
Low-Salt Living

Maggie Coughlin

52 Tips for Low-Salt Living

Copyright © 2019 Maggie Coughlin

Cover design by April Saunders

Wheat Germ LLC
Newnan, GA

ISBN 978-1-945095-28-3

CONTENTS

Huge thanks, as always, to Romily Bernard, dear friend, chosen family, and the best writing partner on earth.

Also to April Saunders, BFF extraordinaire, creative genius, and cover designer nonpareil.

Finally, to Joyce Beverly, who said the magic words "Why aren't you writing a book about this?"

For Clark, for whom I learned it all to begin with.

I always loved your glasses.

INTRODUCTION

"You need to significantly reduce your sodium." Those are not happy words – especially once you start reading labels and measuring milligrams and realizing just how much salt is in virtually everything we eat.

The experts – physicians, nutritionists, etc. – are in kind of a tough position. They have a professional duty (and usually a genuine desire) to keep you as healthy as possible. That generally means transmitting a whole lot of information in a short period of time and it can be hugely overwhelming. They're also understandably torn between urging folks to follow their diets strictly and begging people to at least, for the love of god, cut down on the fast and processed foods. And they don't want to let on that it's going to be a tough adjustment for fear people will be discouraged and give up. Besides, let's be honest, I've yet to meet a nutritionist or a physician that works with diet-restricted patients who *doesn't* eat ridiculously healthy meals themselves. Which is awesome and something we all should aspire to, but just isn't reality for most people facing a major change in diet. If we were all already eating the way they eat, we wouldn't have whatever problem we have now. Short version: the pros are in a tough spot.

I am not. I'm not a nutritionist or a physician or anything vaguely healthcare related at all. I'm just someone who spent most of last year immersed in learning how to make low-salt work on a day-to-day basis. So I have the luxury of telling it like it is – and the real life experience to make specific recommendations you can actually tackle. I also happen to be a professional writer, not a clinician, so I don't have to present all if-thens and whatnot. This is not intended to be a comprehensive book or an exhaustive examination of all things low-sodium or a detailed educational text. It's just supposed to be a helpful – and usable – resource for everyday low-salt living.

That said, because I'm not a doctor or nutritionist, you really do need to run the advice in this book past yours to make sure it fits with your specific combination of conditions. There's a very big difference between reducing salt because your blood pressure is a little high and lowering salt intake because your kidneys have begun to fail. Congestive heart failure, diabetes, and a whole host of other conditions can come into play when we start talking about low-sodium eating. You need to understand what you have and how it works together the best you can. So always consult your doctor before beginning any program, etc. etc.

Full disclosure, I'm not on a medically suggested low-sodium lifestyle myself. Someone who is came into my life and I was cooking for him regularly. Since I quickly discovered that low-salt can be a major adjustment, I decided to put myself on it as well so that my tastebuds would adapt and I'd be better able to look at it as a lifestyle shift. Though we've since parted ways, I've pretty much stuck to the switch. I feel better and taste things differently and the fact is, most people eat far more salt than organizations like the American Heart Association recommend anyway. So even if your doctor hasn't told you to cut the salt, you might want to think about it anyway.

Another note. I sometimes use "salt" and "sodium" interchangeably throughout this book. They really aren't quite the same thing. *Sodium* is a naturally occurring element. It's number 11 on the periodic table, if you're interested. *Salt* is a combination of sodium and chloride. (FYI, sodium chloride on a label is totally salt.) But the vast majority of *sodium* people take in comes through some form of *salt* in food, so that's where most of our focus is going to be.

Finally, I mention a small handful of companies by name throughout this book. Nobody gave me anything to do so. These are just products I have personally found to be worthwhile or that I like using. It doesn't mean they're the only option – or even the one you'll like best.

Okay. Enough intro. Let's get started.

SECTION ONE:
GET YOUR HEAD IN THE GAME

Tip 1: Go ahead and grieve

No, I'm *not* kidding. The accepted standard procedure is to focus on the positive and just get going! And yeah, you've got to do that at some point.

But switching to a low-salt lifestyle is a pretty big change. It affects not only how you eat, but how you shop, how you order in restaurants (and how often you go), and how you think about food. For a lot of people, sharing food is a major component of family and social structure. People talk and bond over food, so any time you have to make a significant change in how you eat, it ripples out into those other areas.

Change is stressful. Period. Even healthy change.

In the case of reducing salt, you're getting something better, good health, but you still have to give something up. You've got to change habits. You may have to give up or reimagine foods that have strong positive associations and memories for you. It's going to take thought and intention and effort. You're going to feel restricted. You may feel envious of friends and family who don't have to follow the same diet or make the same sacrifices. It can feel really unfair. It can be incredibly overwhelming.

All of that is valid.

Let me say that again.

Feeling frustrated and sad and angry and jealous and overwhelmed and whatever else you personally feel is valid. You're allowed to feel it. No one gets to tell you otherwise. They're going to try. Don't accept it. Feel the feelings. Say the things. Go through the grief process of giving up your old lifestyle. Until you do that, you'll never really be free to commit to your new, healthier life.

Grieve first.

Tip 2: Now move forward anyway

I know it's easier said than done. But the reality is that you can't mourn and dwell on the unfairness forever. If you've been told to lower your salt in the early stages of a problem, you need to get ahead of it or it's going to get worse. If you've already let it get worse, you need to start bucking up or it will literally kill you. I realize that sounds harsh. I'm sorry. But it's true.

Side note: if you've already let it get worse, there's zero point in beating yourself up over that fact. You can regret and "if only" all day but you can't change the past. Find a way to accept that you didn't do what you should have done then and start doing it now.

Moving forward doesn't mean you stop feeling the feelings and jump immediately and fully into the new lifestyle with zeal and joy. Most of us can't just flip that switch – and if you wait for it to flip naturally, you're going to end up a whole lot sicker than you are now. Moving forward doesn't mean you won't still be frustrated or angry or sad at times. It just means finding a way to feel the thing, then let it go and focus on the upside.

While I'm not in healthcare, I am credentialed by the International Coaching Federation and I do a fair amount of executive, personal, and leadership coaching, and I've done a ton of change management in my career. What I've learned over many (many) years of coaching and leading through change is that you need a really solid motivation to help you through the rough spots.

"I'm doing it because I have to" or "because the doctor is making me" is not a motivation. You need a clear picture of why you want to be healthy. Maybe it's to see your grandkids get married. Maybe it's so you don't leave your spouse a too-young widow. Maybe it's so you can get irritated over a mistake at work or walk up a flight of stairs without risking a dangerous blood pressure spike. Maybe it's so you can garden more, play with your kids or pets, or just feel less yucky all the time. Maybe it's all of the above.

Figure out what it is for you and make a list or a picture collage and put it somewhere you can look at it when you're struggling. If you feel ridiculous doing it, do it anyway. I don't care who tells you it's silly. It works.

Once you have your motivation firmly in place, mentally commit to making the change. Commit to doing it even when it's hard, even when you're tired, even what you just do not want to. You're going to slip and that's okay, but commit to seeing the slip and recovering.

Falling down matters less than getting back up.

Tip 3: Start retraining your brain

Everything we do begins in the brain. We frequently aren't conscious of that fact – we do a lot of things automatically every day – but it's true. It's also true that neural pathways are a thing. That, in fact, is *how* we manage to do so many things on autopilot each day. Your brain gets used to sending a specific signal in response to a specific situation and eventually you just respond without conscious thought.

This is why the memories associated with places, smells, sounds, and tastes are so strong. We taste the comfort food mom always made us and we feel loved and cared for. We taste a favorite broke-college-kid food and we're right back in those younger, less stress-filled days. Switching to a low-salt lifestyle isn't just about giving up the actual tastes we've gotten used to; it's about finding new ways to trigger the great emotions those tastes bring us. Frankly, that's the harder part – and the part nobody talks about.

If you want to change your actions, you need to change your thoughts. This means changing how you think about your new low-salt life. (Yes, you've heard this before from a thousand health experts: it's not a diet, it's a lifestyle change. This is why they say it.)

Stuff you need to stop saying (and thinking):

- This food is really delicious...for a low-salt meal.
- Don't tell me about the sodium; I want to pretend it's normal food.
- If I follow the rules today and tomorrow, I can "treat" myself on Thursday.
- I'm eating this, but I don't like it.

In all those scenarios, you're telling your brain that eating low-sodium food is bad or abnormal. It's not. It's far healthier and far more natural. It's just different than what we're used to (more on that in the next section). Replace those thoughts and words with alternatives:

- This food is good
- I like that this tastes good *and* is good for me
- I'm being really healthy day-to-day and it's okay if one choice can't be as healthy as I'd like
- I'm eating this because I like feeling healthy

Here's another one that has to go:

- My doctor won't let me eat that.

Your doctor is not the boss of you. You are the boss of you. You can choose to feel like crap, get sicker, and die if you want. Your doctor is an expert advisor whose job is to give you the information, medication, and support you need so you can get and maintain your best possible health. Actually doing it is your job. Take responsibility for it.

On a related note, also ditch "My spouse won't let me eat that." That person is also not the boss of you and also not responsible for "making" you do the right thing, though if you've committed to a shared life, they certainly ought to get some say in the matter. But at the end of the day it's still *your* life. *Your* choice. *Your* responsibility.

Try this instead:

- I'm not going to eat that because I want to live my healthiest life.

Follow it up with the motivations you identified in the last tip.

Get in the habit of reframing how you think and talk about this change. Your sodium intake may be restricted, but you can free your mind.

Tip 4: Take comfort from the fact that you *can* retrain your tastebuds

Salt is everywhere, especially in restaurants and prepared and shelf-stable foods. To be more specific, *too much* salt is everywhere (more on that in the next section). Our tastebuds have thus been trained by a lifetime of eating to register too much salt as the correct amount. So when we cut salt, food suddenly seems bland. It's not really. We just expect more salt and associate higher salt with higher flavor.

Have you ever discovered something you thought was a fact was really an urban myth? Or that the way you've been saying something is incorrect grammar or pronunciation? But when you find out the correct way, it *sounds* wrong because you're so used to hearing it the incorrect way? Same thing. The absurd amount of salt we consume, especially if we eat out a lot or use canned and boxed foods, is incorrect. But we're used to incorrect, so the right amount of salt tastes wrong.

The good news is that your taste receptors really will adapt – and it's actually easier to retrain them than it is to retrain your brain. I went out for a restaurant steak about six months after I'd cut salt to a minimum and could hardly eat it (more about restaurant steaks later). In fact, at this point, most restaurant foods are far too salty for me. Which is, frankly, annoying and a little sad because darn it! I used to love that fettuccine Alfredo and those scrambled eggs. My brain *wants* to love the food still because I have positive memories associated with it. But my tastebuds are over it. So then I feel sad and then I get over it and I end up feeling better. This will happen for you too in time – if you stick with it!

Tip 5: Ask for help

Look, you *can* do this on your own (you can, I swear) but it's unquestionably harder that way. So why would you make an already tough thing harder if you don't have to? If your friends and family love you, they want you to stick around and there's a good chance they'll be on board with helping you be healthy. Does that mean they'll jump into the low-salt life with you? Meh. Maybe, maybe not – even if their doctor has told them the exact same thing. But even if they aren't eating it, they can learn to support you in your journey.

The key here is that you need to figure out how you need to be supported. Do you need accountability? Do you need someone to just listen to you vent when you're frustrated? Is it helpful to try out a new recipe or food together? Do you need help with research? Do you need someone to help you get back up after you slip? Do you need to meet at a park and bring your own food instead of going to a restaurant? Don't assume people know what you need and will respond accordingly. What they would need if the roles were reversed might be very different than what you need and nobody's a mind-reader. Be honest and open with your support system about how you're feeling and what you need. Preferably while you aren't in the grip of frustration or despair because, at those times, you just want it to go away and that's not possible. When everyone is calm and thinking clearly, sit down, talk it out, and come up with a support plan.

If your friends and family can't or don't support you – or if you don't have anyone handy, talk to your doctor, nutritionist, or local hospital or specialty clinic about support groups. The American Heart Association maintains an online network at supportnetwork.heart.org and the American Association of Kidney Patients maintains a list of groups at aakp.org/support-groups. The latter also published a guidebook for support groups if you decide to start your own. These groups can be immensely helpful.

In fact, consider finding a virtual or in-person support group even if your personal network is behind you all the way. I understand the low-salt life because I live it, but I still live it by choice. I can slip up without my ankles swelling, without getting dizzy from rocketing blood pressure, without feeling rotten for days. My emotions surrounding this lifestyle are much different than those of someone on a doctor-prescribed low-sodium plan. The same will be true of the friends and family who support you (and it's important for them to remember this). Having access to people who know exactly what you're going through can be invaluable.

Find them and talk to them.

SECTION TWO:
GET EDUCATED

Tip 6: Accept that there really is way too much salt going on

Seriously. As of the 2015 Dietary Guidelines for Americans (the most recently published as of March 2019), the Food & Drug Administration recommends people who aren't on a low-sodium diet consume less than 2,300 mg per day. People on a low-salt plan are generally told to aim for a max of 1,500 mg. However, the average American, per the FDA, consumes more than 3,400 mg each day. Folks who eat out a lot or use a lot of processed foods tend to get way more than that.

When I first found out about this, I opened my pantry and started looking at labels. I was *horrified.* That can of super healthy, high-fiber organic black beans? Half a day's sodium in one can – for someone who *isn't* supposed to reduce salt! So then I started looking at my favorite "healthy" restaurant dishes. Holy. Mackerel. A shared appetizer, a salad, and an entree? Quite frequently two or three *days'* worth of sodium. And, again, that's for someone who doesn't need to cut back.

The biggest shocker for me, however, was that sodium naturally occurs in food. It makes perfect sense, once you think about it. Sodium is a nutrient just like anything else, so of course it would occur naturally, to some degree. But, in my head, salt was a thing we *add* to food. It never occurred to me that some would already be there. For the most part, the experts aren't worried about the naturally occurring portion. The FDA says about 15% of sodium consumption comes from naturally-occurring minerals in foods. But let's look at some math here:

15% of the average American's actual 3,400 mg consumption is 510. So if you're aiming for 1,500 mg, you're getting a third of that without ever adding salt – or having a manufacturer or restaurant do it for you.

In fact, the American Heart Association would like to see *everyone* reduce sodium to under 1,500 mg per day. Since the key concern with excess sodium is high blood pressure – which can lead to congestive heart failure, kidney damage, and any other number of awful things – this makes sense. Lower sodium = lower BP = lower risk of those other conditions. So you're most likely not the only one in your family, office, or friend group that ought to be cutting back on sodium. You're just the one who's getting it done.

Tip 7: **Know your personal numbers**

Before you get hung up on the 1,500 mg number, talk to your doctor and get the one that's right for you. Don't accept an answer like "just don't eat out so much or add salt to things and you'll be fine." I get why doctors say that; the majority of people who are supposed to be on low-sodium diets are what the healthcare community calls "noncompliant." This is a polite, clinical way of saying they aren't doing what they're supposed to be doing. Often, healthcare providers and nutritionists are just trying desperately to get patients to cut out some of the excess – and to make it as easy as possible for the patient to comply, at least to some degree.

But, at the end of the day, that doesn't really sort the problem. Your blood pressure will just worsen more slowly. You'll live longer, maybe, but the excess salt will still eventually take you out. That's not really what one might call a desired outcome.

So get a hard number – and be careful of assuming the paperwork you've been given will give you the answer. I spent three hours wading through an inch-thick stack of densely-worded material. I found three different numbers for the patient in question's recommended maximum daily sodium intake. They differed by as much as 20%. That's a big range. Get your number – and, again, make sure you understand why it's important for your condition and whether there's anything else you need to be watching for.

Tip 8: Get a visual

Most people are highly visual, but how many people know what 1,500 mg of sodium looks like? Or 2,300 or 3,400, for that matter? The easiest way to get a visual is to go measure out a teaspoon of table salt. Table salt is about 40% sodium and one teaspoon is about 2,300 mg.

Pour that teaspoon into your palm. You'll probably have to cup your hand because it's more than you think. Now look at it and imagine just swallowing all that salt. It's...not a yummy thought. But you're probably taking in way more than that on a daily basis. That's not so yummy either.

You might consider keeping that teaspoon of salt in a clear container where you can see it. It's a pretty good reminder of just how much we oversalt things – and possibly a powerful motivator.

Tip 9: Stop shaking

One piece of advice you'll read over and over again is to take the salt shaker off the table. You'll read it so often you may sprain a muscle from rolling your eyes. It really is a thing you ought to do, though. Instead, add a shaker of garlic (not garlic salt or seasoning, but actual powdered garlic), the pepper mill, or any number of other options (more on spices and flavorings soon).

Besides removing the shaker from the table, you also need to stop, well, *shaking* it. An open-hole salt shaker can dump as much as ⅛ teaspoon or more on your food with each shake. Think I'm exaggerating? Go try it. It's ridiculous.

Ideally, you really shouldn't add salt to your food period, but if you absolutely must, put it in your hand first so you can see and control how much you're really using. If you can't do that for some reason, gently tap the tip of the shaker with your forefinger rather than actually shaking. My grandfather always salted his food this way, a habit he picked up shipboard during WWII, when a lurch of the vessel could catch you mid-shake and pour out far more salt than you'd intended. Turns out it works for low-salt living too.

Tip 10: Understand sodium's role in the body

Like fat, salt is not inherently evil. We all need a certain amount of sodium to be healthy. It helps balance the fluids in your body (which is why you may swell/retain fluid if you consume too much). It also helps your muscles function properly and plays a role in sending impulses through your nervous system.

Sodium's role in fluid balance is why it can contribute to high blood pressure. Too much sodium pulls water into your bloodstream, which drives up your blood pressure. Basically, more fluid has to push through the same sized tubes (your veins and arteries), which means more pressure. That means your heart has to work harder and therefore, over time, wears out more quickly. Because your kidneys are responsible for processing sodium and other nutrients, excess salt (and fluid) can wear them out more quickly too. High blood pressure can wreak havoc on your health in myriad ways.

Bonus zinger: recent research suggests that some people are simply more sensitive to salt than others. Your weight, age, race, gender, and other conditions can make you more susceptible to rises in blood pressure as a result of sodium. That stinks. No question.

However, experts also say many people with high blood pressure don't even know it. The American Heart Association calls it "the silent killer" for that very reason. You do know and that means you can do something about it. That puts you one step ahead.

Tip 11: Understand salt's role in taste

If you remember grade school science class, you'll remember that humans taste five basic flavors: sweetness, sourness, saltiness, bitterness, and umami. Actually, you might not remember that last one; it's been added fairly recently. Umami is basically savory. Bitterness can be tasty or otherwise and it comes from citrus rinds, coffee, unsweetened cocoa, olives, etc. Sourness, in cooking, is often referred to as acidity. It comes from things like citrus fruits, wine, and certain food-safe acids. Sweetness is sweetness and saltiness is saltiness.

The catch here is that pretty much the only thing that tastes like salt is...sodium. Potassium chloride, the primary ingredient in most commercial "salt substitutes," comes sort of close. But, for the most part, salt is salt. This, by the way, is why everyone needs some sodium in their diet; when your saltiness receptor is triggered, it sends out neurotransmitters that trigger reactions in your nerves and muscles (funny how that all works together, huh?)

The point, from a flavor perspective, is that you can't really replace saltiness. You just have to increase the other flavor profiles to compensate. And you do want to replace it. Too often, people just start leaving out the salt and, yeah, stuff then tastes bland. And then you get sad and frustrated and annoyed and binge out on bad stuff. Instead of just leaving out the salt, you need to find other tastes to add so your food is still interesting and flavorful. That's what we'll focus on in the next section.

Salt's unique flavor is the other reason you hear people on low-sodium diets complain that, no matter how good something tastes, it just doesn't taste *the same*. It doesn't. It won't ever. As we said earlier, that can present quite a mental challenge when a flavor is tied to memories and emotion. It's okay to feel sad or disappointed about that. But feel the thing and move forward anyway. One option: be intentional about making new positive memories associated with the new taste.

Tip 12: Understand why restaurants and food manufacturers use so much salt

Short version of the restaurant question: excess salt stimulates the heck out of the saltiness taste receptor, which means you don't notice the lack of other flavors so much.

It's a little more complicated than that, but not much. Part of it, especially in the U.S., is that our tastes are, as discussed earlier, adapted to an absurdly high sodium content. So if it isn't salty, people think it isn't "good." Generally (not always, but generally), the more high-end the restaurant, the more judicious their use of salt. This is one reason fast food is so horrifically sodium-soaked. To tastebuds trained to expect it, a lot of salt covers a lot of culinary sins.

Also applicable to chain restaurants, in particular – and to canned and boxed foods as well – is shelf-life. Salt is perhaps the world's most basic preservative. Long before refrigeration, people salted the bejesus out of meat to keep it from going bad. Then it had to be soaked for hours or days before use to pull the salt out. Food manufacturers still widely use salt as a preservative because it's cheap and hey! it's also "natural." That's why you'll find so much sodium in canned, boxed, and frozen foods – or anything that was prepared from frozen, as many restaurant sauces, soups, and other items are, especially in large chains.

Also, beware the low-fat trap. Want to cover up a reduction of flavor caused by lowering fat content? Add salt! Seriously, that's often how it works. Not always, mind you. Sugar is often used this way as well, and (some) food manufacturers have become more responsible over the years. But still, if you compare the sodium level on a low-fat or fat-free product with its full-fat counterpart, you'll quite often find that lower fat means higher sodium. Always check those labels and think about whether it's really worthwhile.

Tip 13: Know your resources

Your doctors and your nutritionist should be terrific resources for you as you work through this transition. If they aren't, you might need to think about whether they're the right professional for you. If you haven't been assigned a nutritionist, ask for a referral. You can also check with your local hospital to find out what resources they offer to support patients with your condition(s). Your insurance company might also offer literature or other support.

Online, I suggest you bookmark the following:

- Heart.org (American Heart Association)
- Kidney.org (National Kidney Foundation)
- NHLBI.nih.gov (National Heart, Lung, and Blood Institute – you can look for your specific condition or conditions here too)

I also found that both the Cleveland Clinic and the Mayo Clinic had helpful information on their websites.

You can also ask your doctor which other sites have reliable information based on your specific set of conditions. If you're diabetic, for example, you may need to adjust for both sugar and salt, so you'll need to be careful which recipes you follow.

Above all, never be afraid to ask your healthcare team whatever questions you may have. They are there to help you.

SECTION THREE:
EXPAND YOUR FLAVOR TOOLKIT

Tip 14: Research recipes

We're going to talk about some specific options for adding flavor in the next several tips, but it may feel a little overwhelming if you don't cook a lot or if learning to substitute through trial and error sounds way too complicated and time-consuming. The last thing we want to do is overwhelm you more!

The upside is that you don't have to figure it out for yourself. There are dozens of excellent low-sodium cookbooks out there, including a few published by the American Heart Association. You can also find low-sodium recipes on many of the websites listed in Tip 13, and on countless blogs. I personally maintain a Pinterest board just for low-salt living (Pinterest.com/MaggieSheWrote/Low-Salt-Life). If you're on Pinterest, I recommend you do the same.

Side note about Pinterest: if you don't have an account, I urge you to try it out. It's classified as a "social media" platform, but it really isn't. It's basically a search engine (like Google or Safari, etc.) that uses a lot of pictures. I find the results contain a whole lot less junk and way more usable info than traditional search engines. Plus, you can save recipes and other tips you love to your "boards" and add personal notes to yourself for later. Most websites these days give you the option to "pin" directly from their site to your Pinterest boards, and it's super easy to learn and use. To me, it's the same as having a physical binder full of recipes or a folder on my computer – except I can get to it on my phone so I always have access.

If Pinterest just isn't your thing, that's totally cool! Just find a method of collecting and keeping recipes that works for you. You'll feel much more confident and empowered knowing you have that resource to draw from.

YouTube is another excellent place to look for recipes and it can be fun to cook along with the videos. I always feel very Julia Child when I do that. What can I say? We take our joy where we can find it, right?

The point is, you don't have to dive in blind. You can start out with recipes other people have developed and then, as you get more comfortable, you can start learning to modify full-salt recipes and family favorites to work with your new lifestyle. The flavors in this section will help you get started with those substitutions, and many of them are very simple switches you can make as soon as you pop into the grocery and pick a few things up. Some, however, take a bit more experimentation, so if you find yourself getting overwhelmed, go back to existing low-salt recipes. You have plenty of options to choose from!

Tip 15: Behold the power of jalapeno powder

As far as I can tell, the flavor element that chefs call "heat" doesn't correlate directly to one of the body's five taste receptors, but it is a thing nonetheless. It is, in fact, a pretty great thing. Adding heat is a terrific way to offset the removal of salt.

Alas, my personal favorite way of adding heat, hot sauce, is off the table. Hot sauces are almost universally salty. So the day I discovered ground jalapeno on my grocery store shelf was a very good day indeed. Pro tip: not all stores carry it, and those that do usually stock it in the Latin/International/Hispanic/Etc. section rather than with the spices. You can also buy it online. The brand I use is Badia, but there may well be others.

The flavor is very different than, say, red pepper flakes, which we'll talk about in the next tip. And because it's quite finely ground, it blends beautifully into sauces, soups, and other dishes. I use ground jalapeno almost as automatically as I use black pepper now, and I absolutely love it in scrambled eggs and chicken salad. As a bonus, you can sprinkle it on individual servings after cooking so that folks who love hot stuff (me) can enjoy more than folks who just want a hint of heat (virtually everyone else I know).

Do go light-handed the first few times you use ground jalapeno. It's stronger than you think it's going to be and the flavor intensifies *a lot* as it cooks. Start safe and work your way up until you find the right balance for you. This is especially true if you're on a reduced fluid program. The last thing you want is to waste precious ounces of water washing away a too-spicy mouthful.

Tip 16: Play with pepper

Pretty much everyone knows black pepper.
But did you know it comes in several different
grinds? In a nutshell, the most finely ground is
practically a power, while coarse grinds produce
larger flakes. If you have a pepper grinder and
use peppercorns, you may be able to adjust your
grind. But you can also buy pre-ground pepper
in several options.

Why does this matter? Different grinds
offer different flavor intensities and they can
also add texture to a dish. Texture adds interest
– and can help offset the lower salt content.

Red pepper flakes, which you've likely
seen at your favorite pizza place or Italian
restaurant are terrific for adding heat and
texture as well. White pepper is in between
black and red, heat-wise, but the flavor itself is
less complex so you can add heat without
necessarily changing the flavor of your food
overmuch. Green peppercorns have lovely
tartness and a certain freshness other peppers
don't carry. Just make sure you buy them dried
as they often come fresh in brine, which is
essentially salt water. Pink pepper isn't actually
pepper at all; they're berries that happen to
mimic the sharpness of peppercorns. They're

also a bit fruity and floral, so it's quite a different flavor than other peppers. Oddly enough, I like a bit of pink pepper in some desserts. You can also buy multi-color blends in both pre-ground and whole peppercorn forms.

Pepper blends can be fun too, just make sure the spice company doesn't add salt to their blend – or make your own. Lemon pepper, for example, adds both acid and heat as well as several complex flavors and is popular for fish, chicken, and more.

Again, remember that what you're looking to do is add flavor and interest to your food. The mistake most people make is deleting the salt without adding anything new. That's what leads to bland meals, misery, and salt-binging.

Tip 17: Say hello to dried citrus peel

In Tip 11, we talked about the bitterness taste receptor. Remember, citrus peel is one of the foods that trigger that receptor. This makes citrus peel a great addition to dishes because you're specifically stimulating a taste receptor that might not otherwise get attention.

Lemon peel is my personal favorite because it carries the strongest flavor, but you can buy it in orange, lime, and a variety of other options. You can also pick up a lemon zester for a few dollars and add your own.

Later, we're going to talk about salad dressings, but I'll tell you now that one of my favorite prepared dressing alternatives is olive oil + white balsamic vinegar + pepper + garlic + dried lemon peel. I also use lemon peel to add brightness to soups, chicken, fish, and more.

As far as "how much," it's really a question of personal taste. Add a bit and try it. Not there yet? Add a bit more. It's not really that different from salting and peppering your food, it's just that we've all been doing that so long we instinctively know how much to add. Start using citrus peel (and other spices and seasonings) regularly and you'll learn how much you like of those options too.

Tip 18: Don't underestimate onion

Alas, I'm allergic to onions (intolerant, technically, but they're still a bad idea for me). This is a massive shame because, if you can use onion powder, it can really ramp up flavor. Stay away from onion salt, obviously, but have a ball with the powder. Fresh onions are terrific, as well, of course, and different onions carry a whole host of different flavors. Dried onions are also an option when you don't have time to chop. Be careful of jarred or canned onions though, because they tend to use sodium-based preservatives.

Another pro tip: check the Latin/International/Hispanic/etc. section of your store for onion powder. You may find the organic onion powder in this section is far more affordable than the organic version made by major mainstream spice companies!

Tip 19: Go for garlic

I mean, everyone knows this by now, right? Garlic is great. It's low-calorie, is a terrific source of vitamin C, vitamin B6, and manganese, and regular consumption has been tied to reductions in cholesterol and blood pressure.

Beyond that, garlic is delicious, affordable, and easy to use. Thankfully, I can do garlic, even though it's in the same family as onion – and I use it all the time, not just in Italian dishes. I keep powdered and fresh on hand all the time – again, stay away from garlic salt and be careful with prepared jarred garlic. It pairs well with citrus flavors and peppers. In fact, I think it's kind of hard to go wrong unless you get way too heavy-handed.

Tip 20: Cinnamon's not just for sweet stuff

Usually when people think about cinnamon they think about desserts, pastries, coffee and tea drinks, maybe oatmeal. It's actually great for savory dishes too. Spaghetti and other squashes, pork, chicken, lamb – lots of foods can pair well with cinnamon. It's particularly powerful paired with fruits and meats. Cinnamon, apples, and chicken, for example. Spend some time on Pinterest looking for recipes and don't be afraid to experiment.

As a bonus, there's a fair amount of evidence to support the idea that cinnamon is good for reducing cholesterol, blood pressure, and inflammation while helping to balance blood glucose. It's full of antioxidants, too.

Tip 21: Pick up paprika

It always surprises me how many people don't regularly cook with paprika. My great-aunt always added it to her homemade hamburgers and scrambled eggs and I grew up thinking everyone did this. Apparently not.

Like ground jalapeno, paprika comes from a whole pepper. It's a little spicy, and you can buy quite spicy varieties, but the paprika most people purchase is fairly mild. This makes it a good option for people who don't love super hot stuff. Americans are partial to sprinkling it on devilled eggs for color or maybe using it on chicken and in chicken salad, but it's actually terrific with shellfish, rice, and vegetables, and in soups, sauces, and stews.

Do be aware that paprika's flavor is activated during cooking. So if you sprinkle it on cold, it's just going to look pretty. The key is to put it in early and let the heat do its work. Paprika does have a higher sugar content than other peppers, though, so double-check with your doctor or nutritionist to make sure it's a good choice for you.

Tip 22: Explore seasoning blends

If you've been given a packet of reading material from your healthcare provider, it will almost certainly contain a few recipes for seasoning blends you can make at home. If that sounds fun to you, awesome! Have a blast with it! I like to cook, but I don't *love* it and I would rather put my eye out with a rusty spoon than measure and pour a series of powders into a little glass jar. Also, I so don't have time for that.

Enter pre-mixed seasoning blends. You've got to be very careful here, because the vast majority contain salt. In fact, there's a very good chance salt will be first on the ingredient list. This is true whether you're online, in a grocery store, or in a specialty spice shop. Leave the ones that include salt alone. You have no idea how much is in there.

Once upon a time, Mrs. Dash was the go-to for salt-free seasonings. For a lot of people, it still is. I'm personally about 50/50 on which Mrs. Dash products I like and which I don't. More and more, however, major manufacturers and specialty shops alike are expanding their salt-free options.

I, personally, am a Penzey's person. I like pretty much everything about them and I absolutely love their products. They also have frequent specials that allow you to try new things. They have an entire salt-free section on their website, and it's pretty extensive. They aren't the only ones, though, so if you'd rather buy elsewhere you certainly have options, they are just my go-to.

One additional warning about spice blends. If you're nerdy like me, there's nothing more fun than finding a local entrepreneur who custom blends spices and sells them at festivals and such. However, many of them don't label the ingredients because that's their secret blend. Ask about salt before you buy.

What I'm really saying is, if a recipe you love calls for, say, Italian seasoning or taco seasoning, and the brand you usually use contains salt, you *can* find blends that don't. They just might not be in your local grocery store's aisle. You can also find some great salt-free blends that you can use instead of ranch dressing mix on chicken or in a recipe. You just have to try a few and find the ones you like.

Tip 23: Spend some time in the spice aisle

Obviously, this isn't an exhaustive list of all the spices you can use. I use a lot on a regular basis. Dried parsley, oregano, and cilantro. Sage. Cumin. Tarragon. I'm allergic to lemongrass, but it's a really cool thing to learn to use if it won't kill you. I've spent a fair bit of time playing with various options, researching recipes, etc. I've been known to pick up a jar and think "what the heck is this and what do people use it for?" – and then go find out. It's something I like, something interesting to me. It's something you can do, as well, if you want.

You don't have to just wing it though. The internet is a vast source of information on which spices are good with which kinds of food. Look it up. Print it out or pin it to Pinterest. Build yourself a new collection of go-to recipes.

My point is that we're all acclimated to using a lot of salt and therefore not needing too many other flavors. A low-sodium diet is the perfect excuse to start trying out new things and experimenting with unfamiliar flavor profiles. Yes, you're losing salt, but you can gain a whole host of new favorites in the process.

Tip 24: Fruit juices are your friends

Specifically, citrus juices are your friends, though you can play with others as well. Remember in Tip 11, when we said citrus juices spark the sourness taste receptor? That's why it works so well.

Yes, this includes lemon juice, though if you've done any research at all, you've already heard the virtues of lemon extolled ad nauseum. Fact is, it really *is* pretty awesome.

So, however, is lime juice. In fact, I use lime far more than I use lemon. If you like cilantro, the two pair perfectly and can really jazz up chicken and rice. I also use lime in crockpot soups, with spices and oil to dress salads, and in sauces. In most cases, I use recipes I found on Pinterest. If the recipe already included lime juice but also salt, I left out the salt and added a little more lime until it tasted good. If it called for lemon juice, I tried lime. If it didn't call for either, but did call for salt, I used a couple splashes of lime or lemon juice instead.

My other favorite is pineapple juice. Yet again, it's a very different, very distinct flavor and it brings something unique to the table, no pun intended. I like it best with meats and earthy spices like cumin, but play around and see what works for you. Again, you can start with existing recipes and just use pineapple as a replacement – or look for recipes that call for it. Pro tip: buy it in the multi-pack of small cans rather than the big jar. It lasts longer that way. Do be careful with pineapple juice if you're diabetic, though, as it has a much higher sugar content than lemon or lime.

I have friends who cook with grapefruit juice, but it's just not my thing (and if you've had an organ transplant, you most likely can't have it). If you aren't restricted, though, give it a try. It might be exactly what your tastebuds love best.

Tip 25: Reach for the vinegar

True story, when I first moved to Georgia from the Midwest 25 years ago, I went to the fair and asked for vinegar for my fries. Imagine my surprise when, instead of handing over a malt vinegar bottle, the vendor looked at me like I'd lost my marbles and then dug out a giant jug of white vinegar. Can you imagine? Yuck.

The thing is, there are lots and lots of vinegars. Red wine, white wine, apple cider, rice vinegar. All of them can add an intriguing zing to recipes and salads – without the stringency of plain distilled white vinegar.

Balsamic is one of the more popular these days and it comes in both white and dark varieties. It's a great option on salads, but also on chicken and other meats as well. Flavored balsamics are available online and in specialty stores, though you should watch for the higher sugar content that may come with fruit-infused varieties.

Again, I realize I'm not being specific about how much or with what or when. It's honestly such a matter of personal taste and I am really not a recipe creator. This is why I say to search for recipes and acquire cookbooks. They'll get you started and you can go from there. If you know you want to try a white balsamic, for example, search for "white balsamic vinegar recipes" and see what you get. If something looks good, try it!

Tip 26: Experiment with oils

Like vinegars, oils come in a vast array of options. Traditional vegetable and canola oils aside, coconut and olive oils are tremendously popular. Olive oils are also often available infused, which can help cut a few steps out of your cooking process.

But oil options don't stop there. Sesame oil, used frequently in Chinese cooking, carries a distinct flavor, as do nut oils like peanut and almond. Avocado oil is another option, as are flaxseed (just be careful not to overuse or it gets funky fast) and grapeseed. Varying your cooking oils can change up your flavor profile and perk up your tastebuds.

Do make sure to use the right oil for the right purpose, though. Hemp seed oil, for example, is rich and nutty and adds great flavor to finished food, but you wouldn't want to sauté with it. Do a bit of research before you start playing with the less common oils.

Also double-check oils with your doctor or nutritionist. People on renal diets, for example, may be told to avoid avocado because of the high potassium content. Don't assume this means your answer is no. Just double-check before you get too creative.

Tip 27: **Wine your dine**

You've probably been told not to drink, but if you cook with wine, you'll burn off virtually all of the alcohol, which is what usually causes medication interactions and other issues. Sweet wines can also be a bit sugary for diabetics, so watch out for that. Double-check with your doctor to be sure, but if you get a green light, cooking with wine can add nice acidity (sourness taste receptor, remember) to a dish.

Dry reds and whites are best in cream sauces and soups and with meats and some shellfish. Dry nutty wines like marsala can enhance chicken, shrimp, and pork. Rice wine is terrific for marinades and some glazes.

Note that I'm talking about using actual wine from the wine aisle or liquor store here. Most "cooking wines" – the ones in the regular shelf-stable aisles – are loaded with salt. I chucked out my cooking sherry when I discovered it packed 190 mg of sodium in two tablespoons.

If you don't know where to start, look for recipes or cookbooks. I know I've said this over and over already, but it's so important for folks to not get overwhelmed and give up. All of the flavors in these tricks can be great additions to your low-salt life, but you've got to learn to use them in a way that feels comfortable for you.

SECTION FOUR:
KNOW THE TOP RESTAURANT &
PREPPED FOOD PITFALLS

Tip 28: Learn to read labels and nutritional info

Ideally, we're all going to immediately switch to only home-cooked, raw food-based healthy meals as of tomorrow. Realistically? Not gonna happen. Sometimes, you just get stuck with prepared foods. And sometimes you need – or just really want – to eat out. For your own sake, I urge you to do so as little as possible, but I still recommend you learn how to read nutritional labels on food and the nutritional info on restaurant websites (when it's available).

For low-salt lifestyle purposes (if you're diabetic, on a renal diet, or have other dietary restrictions you'll need to look at other things as well), there are two main things to be aware of.

The first is the "low-salt" or "lower sodium" label on many canned products. When you look at the actual numbers, you'll quickly find that these products still have far too much sodium. It's just that their full-salt counterparts have even more. Also, be aware that "no salt added" doesn't mean "no salt." It just means they didn't add any in manufacturing. No salt added chicken broth, for example, typically already has a certain amount of salt in it. That doesn't mean you can't use those no salt added products; just make sure you check the numbers for yourself.

That brings us to the second thing, the amount of sodium in the product itself. Most packages label both the actual amount and the percentage of recommended daily intake. Ignore that percentage number altogether. It probably doesn't apply to you. Just look at how many milligrams – and make sure you note the serving size. Too much of an apparently okay product can shoot you into too much sodium territory quickly.

Remember the daily number your doctor gave you and stick to it as much as possible.

Tip 29: Watch your chicken

Chicken is the healthy animal protein, right? Except...

Some chicken processors inject it with a mixture of salt, water, and other preservatives to keep it fresh longer. A standard serving of chicken that's been treated this way can pack a whopping 400+ mg of sodium, which means you could end up spending a solid 25% - 30% of your daily allowance in one chicken breast – and that's if you add nothing to it. Chicken that hasn't been treated, however, runs more like 70mg of sodium in a 4-ounce serving. Much better.

To make sure you're getting the healthier option, check the nutritional label or look for a notation that says something like "up to 15% chicken broth added." If they've added broth, back away. Unfortunately, this probably means paying a bit more per pound. But remember, that 15% adds volume too. So for every seven pounds of chicken with added broth you buy, you may actually get as little as six pounds of meat.

Tip 30: Can the condiments – but not all of them

Y'all, I like a good barbecue sauce as well as the next person. And we've already discussed my obsession with hot sauce. But prepared condiments, by and large, are just chock full of too much salt, too much sugar, and too many preservatives. It's a sad, sad fact to accept, but we really, really need to do it.

Here's the good news, though: you can find healthier condiments. I'm not sure I'd go so far as to say "healthy," but okay for light use, for most folks. My two go-tos are Beaver brand hot cream horseradish and no salt added Westbrae Natural organic stoneground mustard. The horseradish contains a few things I could live without, but it does only have 20 mg of sodium per teaspoon and it's yummy. The mustard is pretty great, too and it's nothing but vinegar, water, mustard seed, and spices – and there's zero salt! Again, these aren't your only two options. To find healthier alternatives, you'll have to flip over a lot of containers and read the labels. But if you go take a look at the condiment bottles in your refrigerator now, you'll see why it's worth the effort!

You can also replace the flavors some condiments add with other options. Not gonna lie, I love mayo. And the organic brand I buy is actually not so bad salt-wise. But I now use only a little bit on sandwiches – and then sprinkle on a few drops of olive oil or add my low-sodium mustard or horseradish for creaminess. If I'm making chicken salad, which I also love, I cut the mayo in half and replace the rest with avocado. Deviled eggs? Leave out the pickle relish or green olives and use fresh or dried dill instead. Again, always check with your doctor, especially if you have conditions other than high blood pressure, to make sure the substitutions are okay for you.

Tip 31: **Kiss canned soup goodbye**

In fact, most prepared soups have to go, unfortunately, even the ones in restaurants and available hot in your grocery's deli or prepared foods section. The American Heart Association has identified a set of foods they call "The Salty Six" because there's just so very much sodium in them. Prepared soups, especially canned, is one of the six.

I would love to tell you I found a good-tasting, low-sodium commercial option. I didn't. I'm sorry. I make all my soups myself now, mostly in the crockpot. And I'm very, very careful of what goes in them. Alas, this is the best I've got for you on this one. But homemade soups do taste awesome, are frequently freezable, and the house always smells wonderful.

I was able to find several options for no salt added broths that really are low in sodium, and those make good soup bases. Again though, watch for that "lower sodium" label on broths. Lower doesn't necessarily mean low enough.

Tip 32: Approach the deli with caution

Guess what else is on the AHA's Salty Six list? Processed meats and cheeses. Mostly, this means items in the deli – and at your favorite sandwich shop. It also includes bacon, sausage, packaged pepperoni, and more. But one of the big culprits is deli meat because it's so often touted as low-carb and low-cal. And, mostly, it is. Sodium is another story. A 2-ounce serving of meat from the deli can range from 300 mg to 600 mg of salt – or more. Packaged meats are typically even worse.

Cheese...well all cheese is fairly salty. There's no way around it. You'll just have to limit it, which makes me personally quite sad because it's my favorite. That said, Swiss, mozzarella, high quality parmesan, and Monterey Jack tend to be lower in sodium, so opt for those first. Feta, blue, and Edam are notoriously high in salt, while cheddars and others fall somewhere in between.

The good news is that Boar's Head has a whole range of AHA-certified products. The downside is that this only means a serving has less than 480 mg of sodium, which is still pretty dicey if you're on low-sodium. Still, if you're careful, it's something you can put on your list on occasion. Also, however, Boar's Head offers two roast beefs and a turkey that range between 40 mg and 80 mg and that's very doable. I don't particularly like the turkey, to be honest, but a friend of mine loves it, and I do like the roast beefs. Boar's Head also has a provolone that comes in at 140 mg an ounce, a Munster that's just 75, and two Swisses that come in at 35 mg and 60 mg respectively. I like all the cheese options, but the muenster is kind of tough to find in my area.

The point is, you do have options, but you've got to be very, very careful – and very intentional about your choices here.

Tip 33: Beware the bread aisle

Alas, salt is a key component of breads, crackers, and the like. As a result, the total sodium content can add up fast if you're eating much of it. There are several lower sodium options available these days, though. English muffins are typically on the lower sodium side, as are breads made fresh in the bakery.

As far as packaged products go, my favorite is Toufayan Bakeries' Smart Pockets. They come in three or four varieties and only contain 80 mg per pocket. They're flavorful and easy to stuff, and they hold up well.

Unsurprisingly, sandwiches can be a problem sodium-wise. Salty bread + salty condiments + salty deli meats and cheeses = a whole heck of a lot of salt. But if you fill one of these pockets with some of the above very low sodium meats and cheeses, then dress it up with a very low salt mustard or horseradish and add in some veggies, you can have a pretty yummy sandwich. Eggs scrambled with spices and veggies with a bit of Swiss is really good too. Sandwiches are not dead to you. You have options.

On a related note, several cracker companies also offer lower salt options. Just make sure to check the label to verify what that means. If you like matzos (I personally do), you can also find those in low-salt varieties and I don't think they taste much different than the regular ones.

When you're looking at crackers, be sure to compare brands. I was surprised to find that, in several cases, the store brand had less sodium than the equivalent national brand. In fact, I often found that to be the case with shelf-stable goods, especially at Kroger. Oh! And when it comes to bread crumbs, unseasoned panko is by far your best bet.

Tip 34: Pick your pasta carefully

Pasta isn't the worst offender of the sodium world, by any means, but it can get pretty high. This is one of those cases where you just have to check the package and see.

Since I was dealing with both diabetic and salt restrictions last year, I spent some time exploring veggie pastas. Not the ones made by the big, mainstream pasta companies, but those over in the organic section. We liked Explore Cuisine edamame spaghetti which has zero sodium, and several of Cybeles' varieties, which are mostly very low in sodium (under 30 mg/serving). Not all organics (of anything) are made equal though, and even many organic products contain a lot of sodium, so choose wisely by reading the labels. Also be aware that, if you're on a diabetic, heart renal or other diet, some varieties may be off the table for you because of phosphorus, potassium, fat, sugar, etc. As I've said a dozen times already, check in with your doctor or nutritionist to be sure.

The biggest pitfall with pasta, though, is the sauce. Honestly, just stay away from the jarred stuff. We found no good options on that front. Instead, make your own using low-sodium ingredients or go with olive oil and spices for something simpler. No idea where to start with this? I bet you already know what I'm going to say. Pinterest, the internet, and recipe books to the rescue!

Tip 35: Be careful with canned tomatoes

For the most part, I just stay away from canned food, period. I do make two exceptions and this is one. I am flat-out too lazy to make my own sauce from actual fresh tomatoes. I just am. And I've managed to find some viable solutions.

Here's the thing about canned tomato products: you can find a "lower sodium" option at just about any grocery store. But it's still going to have more salt than it ought to. Enter my two favorite stores for low-salt living: Kroger and Sprouts. Kroger, under its Simple Truth brand, stocks no salt added diced and crushed tomatoes. Sprouts has store-brand no salt added versions of diced and crushed tomatoes both, too, but also a no salt added sauce. All of them come in under 25 mg per serving, which is as much as 90% lower than the standard can, and there's not much in any of them other than tomatoes and tomato juice.

I also discovered that tomato paste has only a tiny fraction of the sodium in tomato sauce so, worst case, pick up a can and add water and your own spices.

Of course, if you're less lazy than I am, absolutely make your own from actual fresh tomatoes. And, again, double check with your doc, because tomatoes are on the no-go list for some people.

Tip 36: Count your beans

The other canned item I make exception for is black beans. (They may be out for some folks, so check first.) I absolutely love the things and, for some reason, I can't convince myself to soak them from dry. It may simply be a personal failing, but I'd bet I'm not alone.

As with tomato products, there are plenty of lower sodium options, but they're all still pretty high. Once again, however, Sprouts and Kroger come to the rescue with no salt added versions that cut the full-sodium varieties by 75% or more. Sprouts also has other no salt added canned bean varieties to try.

Tip 37: Pick better butters

I love peanut butter. Seriously, I eat it every single day. When I first got dogs, I became aware of the sugar level in most commercial peanut butters and found an affordable, great-tasting, no-sugar-added alternative. One with only two ingredients. One is peanuts.

Guess what the other one is?

Yep. Salt. Now, the fact is, this particular brand (it's Kroger's natural creamy, in case you're interested) only has 130 mg of sodium per two tablespoons, so it's not really so bad. Most of the national brands aren't much higher, honestly, but I'd just as soon save 10 - 20 mg each day and pay less since I have the option. I also like to pick up no salt added store-ground peanut and almond butters at Sprouts, especially when I catch them on sale. If I can cut 100 mg or more out of my peanut butter each day, well, to me, that's a piece of cheese I get to enjoy. Other stores also grind in-house and offer no salt added varieties, too. Just watch the expiration dates as no-salt versions don't have as long a shelf life and typically need to be refrigerated after opening. And if you're on a low-fat or renal diet, make sure to check with your doctor as you may need to avoid nuts and nut butters.

I also personally detest butter substitutes and only use real butter – when I use it at all. Turns out I actually like baked potatoes and many veggies better with olive oil and spices. If you do use butter, opt for unsalted rather than salted and you'll cut out even more sodium.

Tip 38: Pause over pizza

Remember the Salty Six? Pizza is definitely on that list. Like sandwiches, it makes sense if you think about it: bread, cheese, tomato sauce, and often processed meat. Most of the top offenders piled onto one plate.

Does this mean you have to eliminate pizza entirely? Not necessarily. Just make it at home and watch what you use. Try a lower sodium pita as a base or make your own dough and eliminate as much of the salt as you can. Use fresh mozzarella instead of packaged and make your own sauce from fresh or using one of the no salt added options in Tip 35. Leave off the meat – or use home-cooked chicken (NOT the packaged kind) instead – and load on the spices and fresh veggies. Is it the same as your local pizza parlor or favorite delivery? No. But it can be pretty darn good in its own right and it puts you in complete control.

Tip 39: Think through your tacos

Alas, tacos and burritos are also on the AHA's Salty Six list. Nachos, my personal favorite, aren't on the actual list, but I've got to assume they're included by extension. Since I'd make Americanized Mexican food its own food group if I could, this made me pretty grumpy too. At first.

Again, this is a situation that makes sense. Start flipping over salsa jars and you'll be shocked by most of the sodium levels. Plus there's tortiallas or salty chips/shells and cheese. Most taco seasonings are incredibly high in sodium. And then there's sour cream and black olives and pickled jalapenos and... Yeah, you get the picture. Sodium piled on sodium topped with sodium.

As with pizza, you don't have to give up your favorite flavors. You can find lower sodium tortillas or make your own, and both Publix and Sprouts offer store brand unsalted tortilla chips that are really, really good. There are a few salsas that aren't too bad, and making your own isn't all that arduous. I honestly start with one of the no salt added canned diced tomatoes in Tip 35 and build from there if I don't feel like chopping tomatoes. I happen to like Mrs. Dash's salt-free taco seasoning kicked up with some jalapeno powder, but my writing partner, who hates to cook, makes her own seasoning and says it's not a big deal. I go easy on the cheese, use the lowest sodium Greek yogurt I can find in place of sour cream, and add some extra powdered jalapeno or some fresh in place of the pickled. And then I pile on spinach or lettuce, more fresh tomatoes, and some sautéed mushrooms. Most people can also add onions for even more flavor.

Again, is it the same? No. But these days I actually prefer my nachos over most restaurant versions. As a bonus, build-your-own nachos or individual pizzas are awesome for at-home get-togethers and families because everyone can suit their own tastes with ease.

The thing you always have to remember with this low-salt life is that yes, you're giving something up, but you're getting something, too. And you'll get a whole lot more of it because you're taking care of your health.

Tip 40: Plan ahead for restaurant meals

Read any diet or nutrition book on the planet and you'll find two primary pieces of advice about eating out at restaurants: "don't do it" and "if you must, plan ahead." I tend to agree. Honestly, doing low-sodium at restaurants is just tough. Things you think are healthy turn out to be laden with sodium. Portions are giant. You're happy and chatting with friends and so you tend to overindulge.

That doesn't mean it can't be done – as long as you don't do it often (once or twice a week is often, y'all) and as long as you plan ahead.

The upside is that many chain restaurants now have their full nutrition information on their websites. Most independent restaurants have at least their menus posted online and, if you have a question, you can call and ask. Whenever possible, take a good look through the menu or nutrition information and find the best possible solution.

If there's a restaurant your colleagues, family, or friends constantly want to visit, go ahead and take a look right now. Figure out what you will order next time it comes up. Set yourself up for success.

Tip 41: Don't be afraid or ashamed to ask

I'm always surprised by how many people don't like to ask servers what's in a dish or what preparation methods are used or if they can leave something out. Since I have food allergies, I got used to having to do so young and just don't think about it, I guess. But when I surveyed folks, I found two common responses: they don't want to be a "difficult" customer and they don't want to call attention to their condition.

Frankly, if you walk into a "fast casual" restaurant, it's what it is. There's not likely to be a single thing there that fits with your low-salt life, so asking is kind of pointless. Once you get into other types of restaurants, however, they're used to being asked questions. You aren't demanding unfair attention; you're making sure you have the right information to make the healthiest choice.

As far as advertising your condition, we've already discussed that we all consume way too much sodium. Plus, according to the CDC, about 29% of American adults have high blood pressure. So you're definitely not alone. Illness is also not an indictment of your character, no matter what anyone tells you. The point is that you may be the only one in the restaurant who *actually asks* the chef to prepare your fish without salt, but you're not the only one who *should be asking*. Give yourself props for doing it instead of feeling guilty or embarrassed. I can promise you, based on personal experience, that you'll get used to it.

Tip 42: Look for the least processed options

We've talked about how processed and pre-made foods tend to have the most sodium, so it makes sense to look for menu items that are prepared on site, rather than simply heated up there. This tends to include items without a lot of sauce and with the fewest ingredients. Grilled chicken breasts, whole fish, vegetables, etc. You do, however, have to watch out for marinades, and it's always wise to request that no salt be added during cooking.

Remember also to keep your portions small – just because it's there doesn't mean you have to eat it – and try to leave the complementary bread alone.

Tip 43: Go easy on the salad dressing

If you're looking for the closest thing to natural, salads seem to make a lot of sense. And they do. Except...

If you order a salad with meat, it's likely been marinated in – or cooked with – salt. Also, there are cheese and croutons and bacon bits and olives and, above all, dressing. Prepared dressings are typically full of sodium. Take a look at your favorite chain's nutrition information and flip over that bottle of dressing in your fridge. You'll see what I mean. Restaurant dressings can easily hit 400, 600, or even 1,000 mg or more of sodium for a regular serving.

You do have some options for making restaurant salads work in your low-salt life, though.

- Ask for dressing on the side and dip or use sparingly
- Ask for cheese and other salty toppings on the side – or to be left off entirely
- Bring your own dressing
- Use oil and vinegar (prepared vinaigrette is not the same thing) and add pepper

- Bring your own salt-free seasoning blend to sprinkle on with your oil and vinegar

Many people hesitate over the "bring your own" advice for the same reasons mentioned in Tip 41, but it's really only a big deal if you make a production over it. I personally prefer honey in my coffee over sugar or sweetener, but not everyone offers it, so I carry my own with me. Occasionally someone asks about it but usually no one even bats an eye. If someone who doesn't know about your health condition does ask, and you don't want to get into it, just say you prefer your option to premade dressings. That may not be emotionally true, but I guarantee your organs are happier with the alternative.

Tip 44: Stick a fork in that steak

I cannot grill steak to save my life. Thankfully, I only want one a couple times a year, so I figured it would be no big deal. But when I took that first bite of a restaurant steak after a few months of low-salt living, I felt like I'd licked salt straight from the shaker. When I did some research, I discovered that my steak of choice – a 12 oz. ribeye –packed almost 700 mg of salt. If I were a New York strip person, the same size steak would have been more like 1,700 mg. The numbers at other steakhouses weren't any better – and were often worse. And that was before I even got to the sides.

I also discovered, however, that many restaurants offer options that are far less salty (sometimes only because the portion size is lower). If you plan ahead by researching the restaurant's website and choose low-sodium sides as well, you can come in under 1,000 mg for the whole meal. Is that great? No. And if you're sensitive to sodium, getting that much in one wallop instead of spreading your allowance more evenly throughout the day can really mess with your body.

Side note: restaurant hamburgers are even rougher. Just...don't.

If you love red meat, I'd honestly recommend you find some good salt-free marinade recipes and spice blends and learn how to do it yourself. Of course, red meat has its problems, sodium aside, so check in with your doctor first and cut back as much as you can.

SECTION FIVE:
LEARN TO LIVE WELL IN YOUR NEW
LOW-SALT LIFE

Tip 45: Plan for cravings

Cravings are going to hit. They just are. Even now, nearly a year after I started adjusting to the low-salt lifestyle, I'll get a sudden urge that just has to be scratched. Since everyone really does need a certain amount of sodium in their diet, it's important to make sure your sodium level hasn't dropped too much, so do keep in contact regularly with your doctor.

But if your levels are okay and it's just a craving, there are things you can do to help ease it. My go-to is olives because, at this point, two or three provide enough to fire off my taste receptors. An ounce of cheese will do the trick for me too, without making a huge impact on my daily intake.

Do, however, be careful of indulging these cravings too often, especially in the early days. Your tastebuds are essentially detoxing from years, maybe decades, of salt overuse. They need time to adjust to the new normal or both your taste and your mind will be perpetually stuck in your old life. As much as possible, stick to your new low-sodium plan. But if you have to satisfy a craving, it's better to get a taste of something salty than to binge on a large pizza with pepperoni and extra cheese.

Tip 46: Notice when your tastes start to change – and celebrate

The good news is that your tastes really will start to change. What once seemed barely salted will suddenly taste like a salt lick. Foods you used to love will leave you nauseated or feeling bloated and gross. Don't be surprised or frustrated if your first reaction is sadness or regret. As we've said before, those old foods may have had powerful memories tied to them. What you're really mourning at this point is the feeling you got from eating those foods, not the food itself.

Again, though, you'll also notice you've gained some new tastes. You'll start to notice flavors that were once too subtle to compete with the excess salt. You'll feel better after you eat and that will improve your mood. Once your tastes begin to adapt, you'll find all kinds of upsides. When you do, celebrate! Just not with the favorite food from your old life.

Tip 47: Beware sneaky non-food sodium sources

While most of our daily sodium intake comes from food, sodium hides (sometimes in plain sight) in other places too. Beverages, including protein powders and drinks, can contain a surprising amount of sodium. Milks, even nut milks, contain varying amounts of sodium, some of them rather high.

But you can also absorb salt through your skin, so make sure to ask your doctor about Epsom and other bath salts, salt scrubs, saline nasal sprays, and the like before using them.

And don't forget that all salt, regardless of what color it is or how organic it is or whether it's high grade sea salt, is largely sodium and therefore not your friend if used in excess.

Tip 48: Take it day by day

Converting to a low-salt life is absolutely doable. That doesn't mean it will always be easy. Especially in the beginning, you'll need to take it one day at a time or one meal at a time or one snack at a time. It's okay to be frustrated. I was serious in Tip 1 when I said you're going to grieve. Grief is a process most people don't move through linearly. There will be days it feels like you flat-out can't do this. There will be days you feel like a superstar. There will be days your plans go sideways and everything feels out of control. You *will* get overwhelmed by the mere fact that salt seems to be everywhere you turn (it is). All that is valid. Feel it as you need to, but keep moving forward. It's the only way you're going to get there.

Tip 49: Manage your stress

If you're converting to a low-sodium lifestyle, you almost certainly have high blood pressure – or are at risk of it. Know what else makes BP soar? Stress. And yet, the process of radically changing your eating habits is stressful. All change is stressful, even the most positive change in the world. And the more stress you're under, the harder it is to stick with new habits. It's a vastly unfair cycle I know, but there it is.

Unfortunately, for many of us, eating our favorite foods was our go-to stress reliever. It's time to find a new, healthy replacement. Make time to try out several stress management techniques and find what works for you. Maybe it's a long walk. Maybe it's meditation or listening to music. Maybe, oddly enough, it's the rhythmic chopping of vegetables. Maybe it's some time in the sunshine or playing with your kids or your pets. Read. Write if you get the urge. Draw, paint, put up new crown molding, listen to a podcast. Find things that help you relax. You may just stumble on a new hobby – and make some new friends in the process.

Tip 50: Talk it out when you need to

In case I haven't been brutally honest enough, let me say it one more time: sometimes this process is going to suck. A lot.

And in case I haven't been crystal clear, let me repeat this again too: switching to the low-salt life contains a huge emotional component that people vastly underestimate – and frequently do not deal with.

You need someone you can talk to – vent to, cry to, whine to, whatever – when it gets tough. Someone who will listen without judging, sympathize without enabling your (understandable and virtually inevitable) urges to veer wildly off course. Find your person (or people), whether it's a friend, a partner, a family member, or support group.

If you find yourself continuously struggling, don't hesitate to talk with a faith leader or professional counselor. You went to a doctor to get your physical health sorted. Seeing a professional to help sort the emotions that come with it is no different. It's all a part of managing your health and being the healthiest you possible.

Tip 51: Remember why you're doing this

When your motivation flags – and it will – go back to your why. Why do you want to be healthier? Why do you want to feel better? Why do you want to live longer? Who loves you? Who needs you? Who values having you around?

What do you love doing and want to do more of? Where do you want to visit – or go back to? What do you still want to try or accomplish or learn? Who do you want more time with?

Never lose sight of the big why. Your *why* gives *what* you do meaning. Your why makes the effort worthwhile.

Tip 52: Share your knowledge

You're going to learn a lot in this journey. At moments, it will feel as though you've learned far too much and you'll wish you could un-know some of the things you've discovered. But everything you learn has value. It can help someone else become a little more informed, make their switch to low-salt living a little easier, make them feel a little less alone.

As you learn, share. Let people into your world. They can help you better that way and there's a good chance you'll help them, too. If their doctor has never told them to lower their salt intake, I can almost guarantee they have no idea how much sodium is hiding where they'd least expect to find it. They have no idea how much they're taking in – and what it can do to them. You *do* know and you can pass it along.

Sharing what you've learned with others will also reinforce it in your mind and help you stay committed when it gets tough. Gradually, low-salt living will start to feel less like some weird, burdensome, abnormal thing you're stuck doing and more like what it really is: a positive reset to what normal ought to be.

Eventually low-salt living will just be... living.

WEBSITES IN THIS BOOK

Resources
Heart.org (American Heart Association)
Kidney.org (National Kidney Foundation)
NHLBI.nih.gov (National Heart, Lung, & Blood)
FDA.gov/food (U.S. Food & Drug Admin.)
AAKP.org (American Assoc. of Kidney Patients)
MayoClinic.org
ClevelandClinic.org
Pinterest.com

Products & Stores
Penzeys.com
MrsDash.com
Kroger.com
Sprouts.com
Publix.com
BoarsHead.com
BadiaSpices.com
BeavertonFoods.com
Westbrae.com
Toufayan.com
ExploreCuisine.com
CybelesFreeToEat.com

My Pinterest Board:
Pinterest.com/MaggieSheWrote/Low-Salt-Life

ABOUT THE AUTHOR

Maggie is a communications trainer, professional strategist, speaker, coach, and writer. Also a dog schmuck, nacho connoisseur, DIY enthusiast, and perpetual student. She loves discovering how to make life and everything in it work better with less stress – and then sharing what she learns.

Find more of Maggie's books on random topics at WheatGermStrategy.com

NOTES:

www.ingramcontent.com/pod-product-compliance
Lightning Source LLC
Chambersburg PA
CBHW050534280326
41933CB00011B/1586